# The Library of Sexual Health™

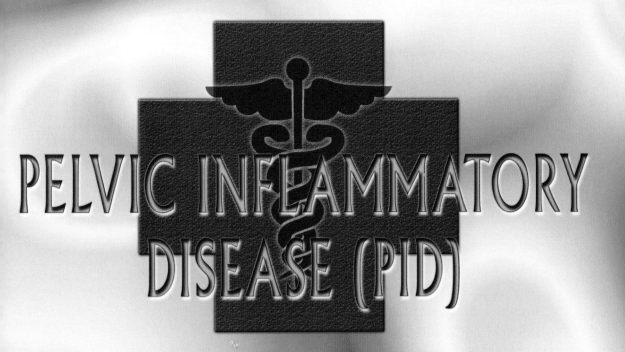

# PELVIC INFLAMMATORY DISEASE (PID)

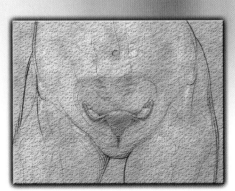

## MICHAEL R. WILSON

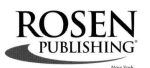

ROSEN
PUBLISHING®

New York

618.1
WIL

Published in 2009 by The Rosen Publishing Group, Inc.
29 East 21st Street, New York, NY 10010

**Library of Congress Cataloging-in-Publication Data**

Wilson, Michael R., 1967–
Pelvic inflammatory disease / Michael R. Wilson.—1st ed.
    p. cm.—(the library of sexual health)
Includes bibliographical references and index.
ISBN-13: 978-1-4358-5059-0 (library binding)
1. Pelvic inflammatory disease—Popular works. I. Title.
RG411.W55 2009
618.1—dc22

                                                                    2008006854


*Manufactured in Malaysia*

3/10
Rosen
@ 21.95

# CONTENTS

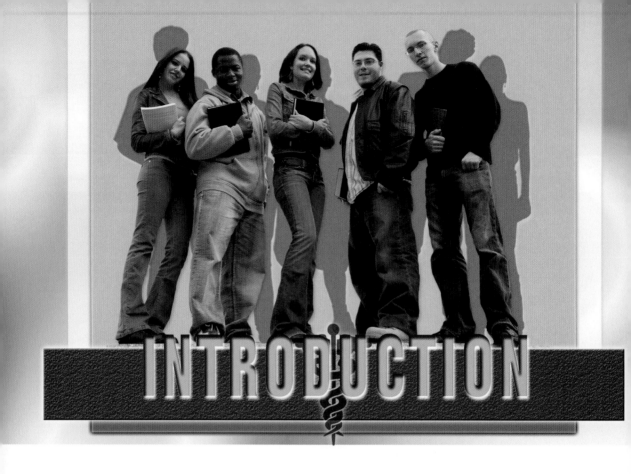

# INTRODUCTION

This book is about pelvic inflammatory disease, or PID, an infection that occurs in a woman's reproductive system. It's usually the result of a sexually transmitted disease (STD), most commonly gonorrhea or chlamydia. A woman with PID is at risk of harm to the organs in her pelvic area. These organs include the uterus, ovaries, and fallopian tubes, all of which are critically important in normal sexual reproduction. Without properly functioning reproductive organs, a woman may find it impossible to have children.

Not all cases of PID lead to serious complications, but some do. Often the disease goes undiagnosed. A woman may notice minor symptoms such as pain and nausea but may think those symptoms are a result of something else, perhaps normal discomfort associated with her period. In some cases, the symptoms will disappear and never return. In others, they'll grow progressively worse and eventually require treatment. Women with severe PID sometimes require hospital stays for intravenous antibiotics. In rare cases, a woman may need surgery.

PID is a complicated subject but so, too, is sexual health. The human body is an intricate composition of

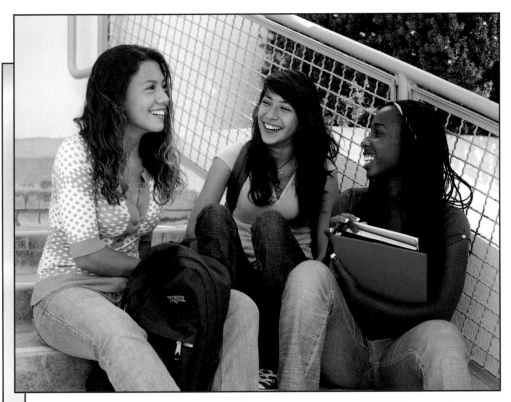

It's great to have friends to talk to about your interests and challenges. Open conversation about sex and relationships is an important part of a healthy lifestyle.

anatomic parts—bones, muscles, organs, and highly specialized tissue. There are countless things that can, and do, go wrong with the body. Many of these things can influence sexual health, even if they're not directly related to a person's sexual organs or reproduction.

This book provides an overview of PID—what it is; the problems associated with it; and how it can be prevented, diagnosed, and treated. It also discusses the many physical, environmental, and social factors that can lead to PID specifically and poor sexual health in general. This book suggests ways people can cope with the disease, and it includes a final section that looks to the future. What are health professionals doing now that may change the way we look at PID ten, twenty, or a hundred years from now? And what good decisions can you make to remain PID-free?

How you use this book is up to you. You may find it helpful if you're doing research for a school report. Maybe you're looking for information to use in your own life or for ideas on how you can help a friend. Whatever the case, be sure to check out the additional resources listed at the end of the book. These books, Web sites, organizations, and other references, taken together, may serve as a complete source of all things related to PID and sexual health. If this book sparks your interest, then use it as a launching point for further investigation.

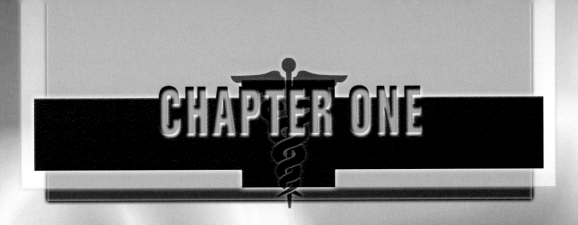

# CHAPTER ONE

# About PID

W e've already mentioned that PID is a disease that occurs in women and can lead to additional problems in the reproductive system. But what exactly does it do? Why is PID so dangerous, and how does it harm the body? How would a woman know she has it, and not some other health problem? This chapter will tackle those questions and more.

## WHAT IS PID?

Pelvic inflammatory disease is irritation of the reproductive organs caused by an infection. An infection is a condition that occurs in the body when pathogenic (disease-causing) germs that aren't supposed to be there invade, multiply, and spread. In some cases, infections do very little harm. A sinus infection, for instance, might make you feel sick for a few days, but usually that's about it. In other cases, infections can be extremely dangerous, even deadly. Infection with human immunodeficiency virus (HIV), for example, can lead to acquired immunodeficiency syndrome (AIDS).

PID occurs when bacteria enter a woman's body through the vagina and migrate upward into her pelvic area and infect one or more of her reproductive system organs. (See diagram on page 10.) It's often said that PID begins in the lower reproductive tract (the vagina and cervix) and spreads to the upper reproductive tract (the uterus, fallopian tubes, and ovaries).

## PID AND SEXUALLY TRANSMITTED DISEASES

Many different kinds of bacteria can cause PID. The most common are *Neisseria gonorrhoeae* and *Chlamydia trachomatis*. PID is not considered a sexually transmitted disease (STD). However, both the *Neisseria gonorrhoeae* and *Chlamydia trachomatis* bacteria are responsible for STDs—gonorrhea and chlamydia, respectively.

Gonorrhea and chlamydia can be contracted through sexual contact with an infected person. Carried in semen and vaginal fluids, *Neisseria gonorrhoeae* and *Chlamydia trachomatis* are spread upon contact with the vagina, urethra, or anus. If chlamydia or gonorrhea bacteria enter the vagina, they can cause PID by spreading upward from there into the reproductive tract.

Bacteria are living organisms. They move around in the body looking for food in the form of sugars. They also reproduce and multiply, spreading rapidly to surrounding body tissues and causing irritation, inflammation, and other damage.

In the case of PID, inflammation and scarring are the most serious problems. When pathogenic organisms invade the body, inflammation is a natural reaction. Inflammation is swelling that occurs as fluid and blood accumulates in tissue. The bacterial infection leads to inflammation of the uterus, fallopian tubes, ovaries, and/or other tissues of the reproductive tract.

Inflammation of the fallopian tubes is also called salpingitis. Endometritis is inflammation of the endometrium, which is the lining of the uterus. Pelvic peritonitis is inflammation of the interior abdomen—the area that surrounds the reproductive tract. Chronic, recurring inflammation can lead to permanent, painful scarring as the body tries to heal itself by replacing damaged tissue with fibrous scar tissue. Scarring within the fallopian tubes may result in infertility, which is the inability to get pregnant.

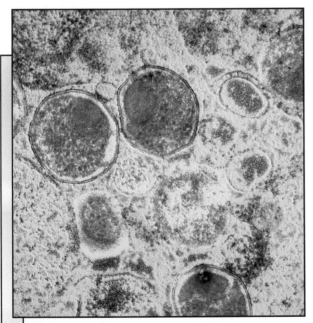

Bacteria such as *Chlamydia* (pink spheres) are microscopic organisms that can invade cells and cause conditions including PID.

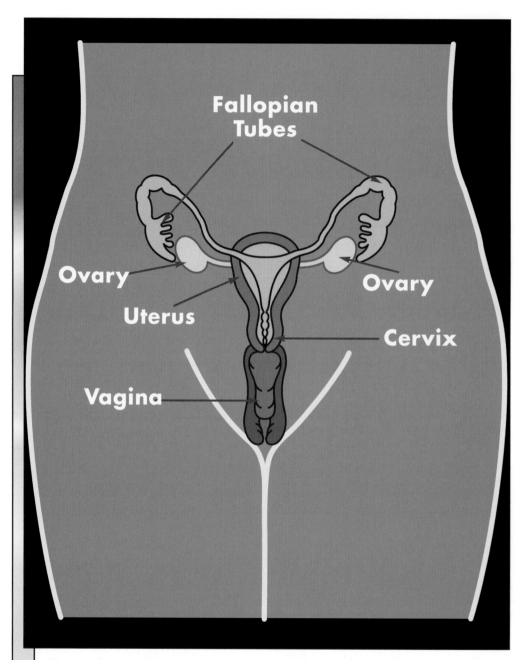

The female reproductive tract is located in the pelvis. It includes the vagina, cervix, and uterus, as well as the ovaries and fallopian tubes.

## A CLOSER LOOK AT THE FEMALE REPRODUCTIVE ORGANS

Of course, in order to fully understand pelvic inflammatory disease, you should first have a basic understanding of female pelvic anatomy. The walnut-sized, oval-shaped ovaries are where eggs are produced. The two fallopian tubes provide a three- or four-inch path through which eggs (ova) can travel on their journey from the ovaries to the uterus. The uterus, also known as the womb, is the largest organ of the female reproductive tract. Its primary function is to house and nourish a fertilized egg (ovum) as it develops from an embryo into a fetus. It does this with help from the nutrient-rich endometrium—the uterine lining—where the egg is implanted. The lower end of the uterus includes a narrow opening called the cervix. The cervix produces mucus that under normal circumstances serves as an adequate barrier to entry for disease-causing organisms. The cervix connects the uterus to the top of the vagina. At childbirth, the infant is pushed through the cervix and through the vagina.

## WHO'S AT RISK?

PID is one of the most serious and common complications experienced by women with STDs. According to the U.S. Centers for Disease Control and Prevention (CDC), more than a million women now seek treatment for PID every year in the United States alone. Many more go untreated

# Sexual Education

According to the U.S. Centers for Disease Control and Prevention (CDC), youth aged ten to nineteen years old, both guys and girls, contract a total of three million STDs every year. The list of STDs includes HIV/AIDS, which almost everyone knows about, but it also includes more common diseases such as gonorrhea, chlamydia, hepatitis B, syphilis, genital warts and genital herpes, bacterial vaginosis, and trichomoniasis.

Chlamydia is a common bacterial STD. Studies show that 40 percent of all chlamydia cases occur among people between the ages of fifteen and nineteen. Girls in the same age group also have the highest rates of gonorrhea. Researchers say too few young women know much about prevention, symptoms, and potential health consequences of individual STDs, and that's a serious issue. "For some of these diseases, they're treatable and curable, but not all are so benign [harmless]," says Julie Downs, Ph.D., the lead scientist in a study on the subject. "If you learn about an incurable disease like genital herpes only after you get it, then it's too late. And even for some of the curable ones, if you don't know enough to recognize symptoms and go to a doctor right away, you're at risk for long-term consequences." Untreated chlamydia or gonorrhea, for example, can lead to PID, which in turn can cause infertility in women. These diseases can also cause infertility in men.

Symptoms associated with STDs are not pleasant. For women with chlamydia and gonorrhea, for example, symptoms include irritation or itching, pain during urination, irregular vaginal bleeding, abnormal vaginal discharge, lower abdominal pain or lower back pain, a high fever, and/or nausea.

When it comes to prevention, says Downs, it's important to realize you can get an STD the very first time you have sex. "Know your partner, and ask them [sic] if they've been tested. If you then decide to have sex, use protection." In terms of STD information and resources, Downs says it's up to the individual to pick up where health class leaves off. "If you have a good relationship with your doctor and can ask your doctor questions, that's a good source of information. Your parents might not really know that much about STDs, but just talking with them about it can be good." Also talk to your friends. You never know—someone else might know more than you!

because they are asymptomatic—they have the disease, but for one reason or another, they show no symptoms and thus don't know they're infected. Of those who are treated for PID each year, up to 200,000 require hospitalization. Also, in many countries outside the United States, especially in the developing world, PID is a common and serious problem. Researchers have studied PID patient populations to determine who gets PID most often. They found that PID is more common in teenage girls than in adults. In fact, an estimated one in eight sexually active adolescent girls develops PID before the age of twenty. Researchers have also found PID is more common in African American women than Asian, Hispanic, or white women. Those most likely to get PID are women who have had an STD. Women with STDs, in turn, are usually younger than twenty-five years old, are sexually active, and have had more than one sex partner. Low socioeconomic status (poverty) is another indicator of risk.

Another group at higher risk for the disease than the general population are women who douche. Douching involves either rinsing or spraying water into the vagina in order to clean it. A variety of devices, including syringes, bags, and other instruments, can be used to douche. Douching disturbs the population of natural microorganisms present in the vagina and can also send harmful bacteria through the cervix and into the uterus, where they are more likely to cause diseases such as PID. Most medical experts do not recommend douching as a means of cleaning the vagina.

An intrauterine device (IUD) is an instrument placed inside the uterus as a form of birth control. Studies have shown that use of IUDs increases incidence of PID when a woman already has a sexually transmitted disease. This is because during insertion of the IUD, there is a possibility that harmful bacteria can be pushed into the vagina. For this reason, women who use these devices should be tested for STDs before their IUDs are inserted. It's not the IUD itself that causes PID; it's the bacteria that may already be present in the reproductive tract.

Several other social and lifestyle factors may increase a woman's risk of contracting PID. Women who smoke, abuse alcohol and drugs, or have multiple sex partners have an increased chance of getting PID. Women who undergo a medically induced abortion have been shown to be at slightly higher risk of getting PID as well. The procedure may expose the upper reproductive tract to pathogenic bacteria residing in the vagina or cervix.

Unfortunately, many women with PID get treatment for the disease only when it's too late. More than 100,000 U.S. women become infertile each year because of PID. In fact, at least 15 percent of infertile American women became so because of damage to their fallopian tubes caused by PID.

## Signs and Symptoms

The signs and symptoms of PID are often hard to recognize.

If they look like those of some other medical condition, then the symptoms may go untreated. Some cases are outwardly mild, while serious damage is taking place inside the reproductive tract. It's a good idea for all women, and sexually active women especially, to know how to recognize even the slightest sign of PID.

PID signs and symptoms vary and depend on the

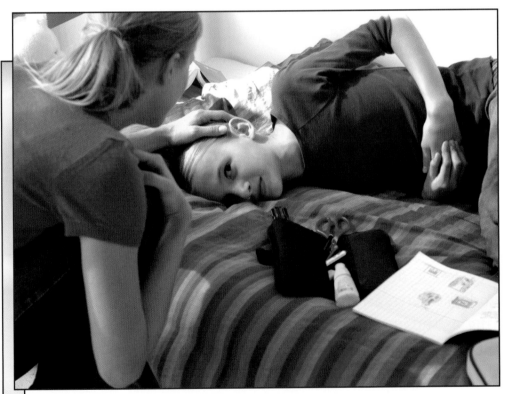

Abdominal pain different from menstrual cramps is one of the symptoms of PID. It's important to seek medical help right away if PID is suspected.

individual, the severity of the disease, and the stage of the disease. The most common symptom of PID is dull pain and tenderness in the lower abdomen. This may be accompanied by fever, abnormal and foul-smelling vaginal discharge (mucus and/or pus), pain during intercourse or with urination, and irregular menstrual bleeding. In rare cases, some women may experience pain in their right upper abdomen. When this pain does occur, it is often sudden and severe and due to involvement of the liver.

In some cases, there are no symptoms at all. When this happens, the woman is at serious risk, as the organ damage taking place inside may be irreparable.

## COMPLICATIONS

Fortunately for most women with PID, the disease can be effectively treated if it is diagnosed and treated early. Left untreated, however, PID can result in a number of serious complications.

Problems arise when the bacteria causing PID are allowed to migrate to the fallopian tubes. When this happens, the damage caused by the bacterial infiltration can lead to the development of scar tissue. Scar tissue is stiff and obtrusive and prevents normal processes from occurring as they should. When present in a woman's fallopian tubes, scar tissue can block her eggs from traveling through the tubes to the uterus. If the tubes are totally blocked, then fertilization becomes impossible. Infertility occurs in

15 to 20 percent of women with PID. The more times a woman has PID, the more likely she is to become infertile due to accumulated scar tissue.

Another complication of PID is ectopic pregnancy. Ectopic, or tubal, pregnancy occurs when a fertilized egg makes it partway through a fallopian tube before becoming blocked. The embryo then lodges in the tube and grows as it would in the uterus. If the ectopic pregnancy isn't removed, then it can grow to a size that causes the fallopian tube to rupture. Pain, internal bleeding, and death may result. Ectopic pregnancy occurs in approximately 10 percent of women who have experienced multiple episodes of PID.

Yet another serious complication of PID is chronic pelvic pain. Chronic pain is pain that won't go away for months or years. Chronic pain, like other complications from PID, becomes more likely with repeated episodes of the disease. It has been shown that women who have had PID multiple times have an 18 percent chance of developing chronic pain.

A history of PID leaves a person at greater risk for future infection from non-STD bacteria. This means it's easier to get the disease again. It's important, therefore, for any woman who has had PID, even if it's cured, to receive regular monitoring for the disease from an experienced health care professional.

Women rarely die from PID. Death can occur, however

(an estimated 150 women do die from PID complications each year), especially if an infection goes untreated or there's a serious complication such as the rupture of a fallopian tube or of a pus-filled abscess within the abdominal cavity.

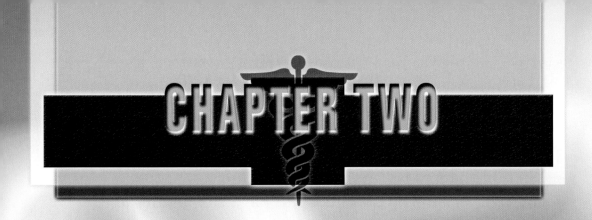

# CHAPTER TWO

# Prevention

T he best way for a woman to protect herself against PID is to protect herself from sexually transmitted diseases. If she does contract an STD, then she should seek treatment immediately.

## RISKY BUSINESS

Because PID is most often caused by the STDs chlamydia and gonorrhea, it only makes sense that the best way to avoid PID is to avoid contracting these and other STDs. One surefire way to stay STD-free is by avoiding any type of sexual contact with another person. A person who chooses to be abstinent decides not to have sexual intercourse. For many teens, abstinence is an easy decision. They're not ready for sex, don't want to have sex, and therefore don't have sex. For others, it's a little more complicated. There are some teens who feel pressure to have sex from friends and peers. Others may want to have sex but are pressured not to by parents, clergy, or teachers.

Still others just aren't even thinking about sex. They probably will someday, but for whatever reason, sex just isn't on their radar. And that's just fine.

For those who do choose to have sex, at any age, safer sex requires using a condom every time. Latex male condoms, unlike oral forms of birth control such as the Pill, not only prevent unwanted pregnancies, they also greatly reduce one's chances of contracting an STD. They serve as a physical barrier between the penis and the vagina during intercourse. This barrier prevents passage of semen as well as the various bacteria and viruses associated with STDs.

Sexually active people should have just one sex partner whom they know to be STD-free. This can be accomplished through simple STD testing at a medical clinic. Once it's certain that both partners are free of STDs, safer sex between them is possible through use of a condom and by maintaining a

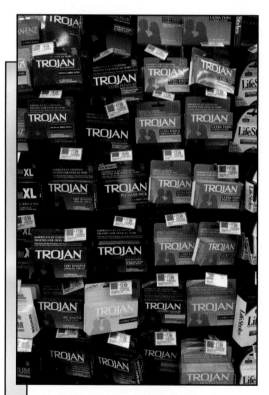

Sexually active individuals should use condoms every time that they have sex. A condom is a means of birth control that also offers some protection against STD infection.

mutually monogamous (one partner only) relationship. Having sex with multiple partners greatly increases the chances of contracting an STD, which, in turn, makes it more likely that the female partner will get PID.

## The Importance of Health Screenings

Studies have shown that routine screening for chlamydia infections in women significantly reduces the risk of PID. The CDC recommends that sexually active women aged twenty-five and younger be screened at least once a year for chlamydia, even if they show no symptoms of the disease. Annual tests are also recommended for older women at high risk for STD infection, for instance those with new or multiple sex partners. Pregnant women should also be tested for STDs, as these can cause serious problems for the babies. In some cases, more frequent screening may be necessary. Women should consult their health care provider to determine exactly how often they should be screened.

Women who are screened and treated for chlamydia before they show symptoms of the disease are nearly 60 percent less likely than unscreened women to develop PID. Without treatment, 20 to 40 percent of women with chlamydia and 10 to 40 percent of those with gonorrhea develop PID.

Regular screening for other STDs is also recommended. The earlier one knows he or she has an STD, the sooner treatment can begin, potentially avoiding more serious

# Chlamydia

Hundreds of thousands of people around the world contract STDs every day. Many of these people are lucky and are treated and cured. Others are not. Of all the countries in the industrialized world, the United States has the highest rate of STD infection. The American Social Health Association (ASHA) estimates that nineteen million new STD cases occur annually in the United States. That number is rising each year, unfortunately.

Among the most common STDs in America is chlamydia. Both men and women can contract chlamydia, and serious complications can arise in either sex, often before symptoms of the disease are even noticed. Chlamydia infections have been on the rise for the last ten years. According to the CDC, in 2004, there were 929,462 reported cases of the disease, an increase of almost 6 percent over 2003. Between 2000 and 2004, the chlamydia infection rate in men increased by almost 48 percent; over the same period of time, it increased by about 22 percent among women. For women, the highest infection rates occur among African Americans, who are more than seven times as likely to report chlamydia than whites, and among those fifteen to twenty-four years old. Among men, those aged twenty to twenty-four are most likely to report the disease. African American men are eleven times more likely to report infection than white men.

Up to 75 percent of women and 50 percent of men with chlamydia show no symptoms of the disease. When symptoms do occur, they typically show up within one to three weeks of infection. One of the most obvious signs is a mucus or pus discharge from the penis or vagina. Pain during urination is also common.

New mothers may pass chlamydia to their newborns when the babies come in contact with vaginal fluids during birth. In men, untreated chlamydia may lead to fever, swelling, and a painful penile discharge, all signs of epididymitis, an inflammatory condition in the region around the testes that can cause sterility. Both men and women are also susceptible to chlamydia infection of the throat or rectum via oral or anal sexual contact.

Fortunately for those with chlamydia, screening for the disease is easy and effective. All it requires is a simple swab collection of fluid from the vagina or penis. The fluid is then sent to a lab for testing for the *Chlamydia* bacterium. Tests may also be conducted on urine samples. Health experts now recommend that sexually active teens receive chlamydia screenings twice a year.

A positive test for chlamydia does not spell doom for the patient. The disease is curable with antibiotics.

complications. Early detection should also keep the person from unwittingly passing the disease to someone else.

A woman who is treated for PID and then goes back to her original disease-carrying sex partner may contract the disease again. Chances are good that her partner is the source of the bacteria that caused the infection in the first place. Women who have had PID, therefore, should ask their sex partners to go to a health clinic and be screened for STDs. If they are then found to have an STD such as chlamydia or gonorrhea, they should be treated—and shown to be disease-free—before having sex again. Doing so also helps prevent the spread of the STD (and potentially PID) to future partners of the infected person. Treating just one person isn't enough; the partner also has to be treated to prevent reinfection with STDs.

In many cases, the sex partner of a woman diagnosed with PID will show no symptoms of a sexually transmitted disease. That doesn't mean he or she doesn't have one.

Anyone who has had sex with a woman who has PID should be screened for STDs. It's the safe and responsible thing to do.

## TALK TO YOUR DOCTOR

One great resource for learning more about sexually transmitted diseases, their prevention, and their potential health consequences is your health care provider. You can ask a doctor anything you want during a routine checkup, and you shouldn't be embarrassed. Doctors are used to this kind of stuff. They deal with it every day, and they also maintain confidentiality.

Of course, talking to your doctor is easier said than done. It takes commitment to develop a strong and open relationship with your health care provider. One study found that more than 50 percent of teens are unlikely to talk with their doctors about STDs or other sexual problems. In most cases, they say, the

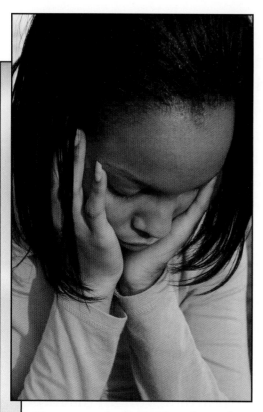

It's not easy dealing with a physical illness such as PID. You may find yourself feeling angry, sad, or embarrassed to talk about it.

subject is just too awkward, especially if there's a parent in the room. Most doctors tend to interview and examine teens alone without a parent in the room, though, to give privacy and to facilitate an open, honest medical relationship.

One way to make things easier is to do some research ahead of time. Get online or go to the library and see what you can learn there first. Then, when you see your doctor, you can ask for more detailed information. To keep it private, ask your parents to stay outside. They'll understand. They've probably been through similar situations when they were kids.

If you suspect that you might have PID, then it's important to see your doctor right away and to be completely honest about your symptoms and your sexual history. Physicians are most effective when they have all the information they need right in front of them. Hiding anything can be dangerous to your health.

## EDUCATION AND AWARENESS

Sometimes, the best way to prevent unwanted infections is through education. The more you know and understand about STDs and how they can lead to complications such as PID, the more likely it is you will take the steps to avoid them.

Reading this book is one way to start. Doing further research—in textbooks, online, or in the classroom—is a good next step. It's important to learn to recognize the symptoms of STDs in general and PID in particular. A woman who

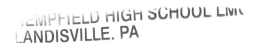

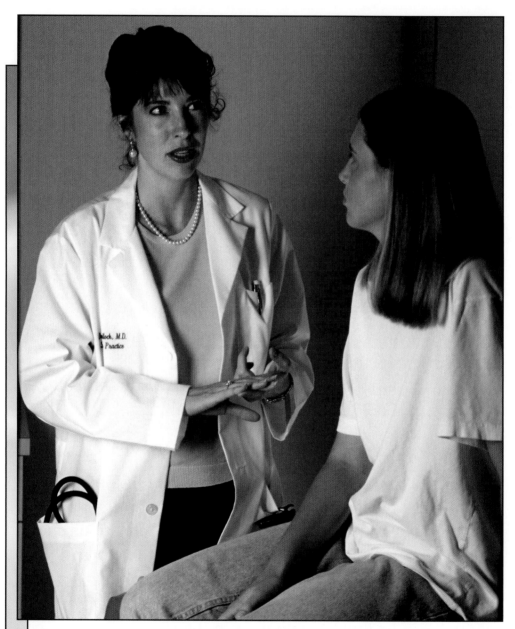

A positive diagnosis of PID is not the end of the world. Treatment for the disease is often effective, especially when it's caught early.

knows what to look for can contact a doctor right away as soon as she suspects possible infection. The sooner she seeks help, the better off she will be.

Early symptoms of STD infection include sores on the genitals, odorous vaginal discharge, burning during urination, and abnormal bleeding. A woman who experiences any of these signs or symptoms should see her health care provider right away. She should also stop having sex and notify her partner (or partners). Needless to say, those partners should immediately go to their health care providers as well.

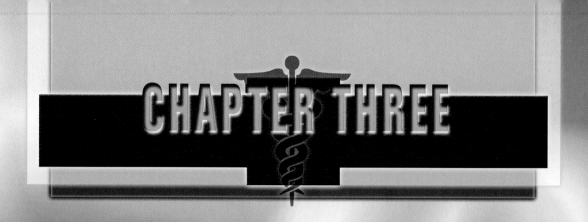

# CHAPTER THREE

# Detection and Treatment

One of the biggest problems with pelvic inflammatory disease is detection. When it's just starting out, the signs and symptoms are so vague and difficult to recognize that they're often mistaken for something else. Even experienced health care providers can have a hard time recognizing the early signs of PID. For this reason, PID often goes undetected at first. Early detection, however, is the key to preventing serious complications such as infertility or chronic pelvic pain.

## FIRST STEPS

If a woman walks into her doctor's office complaining of stomach or lower abdominal pain, the physician may suspect PID. The doctor will typically proceed with a standard physical exam, including a pelvic exam, feeling carefully to locate tender spots and painful areas in the abdomen, cervix, uterus, and ovaries, checking for abnormal vaginal or cervical fluids, and taking the patient's temperature to see if there's a fever. The doctor will check

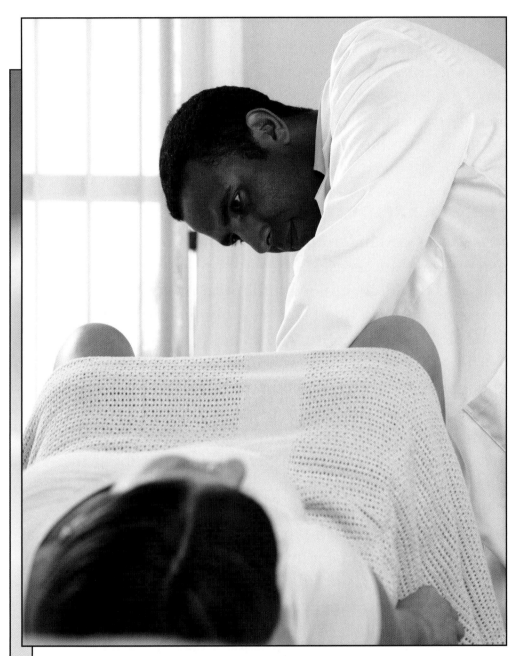

This doctor is taking a sample of cells from a woman's vagina in order to test it for signs of PID. The sample will be examined in a laboratory.

for masses near the ovaries and fallopian tubes and may test for a urinary tract infection (UTI). The doctor may also look for signs of gonorrhea or chlamydia, especially if the woman is sexually active. A pregnancy test should also be done. In the end, the doctor will consider the entire picture before diagnosing PID and making the decision to treat.

## FURTHER EXPLORATION

Sometimes, a standard physical exam is not sufficient for diagnosis. In such cases, laboratory tests may be useful. Lab tests can determine whether the infection is due to the same bacteria that cause chlamydia or gonorrhea, for example. Testing might include looking at blood samples or the swabbing of vaginal and cervical fluids. An endometrial biopsy entails the removal of small portions of the endometrium for analysis. A pelvic ultrasound (sonogram) may also be useful to obtain an image of the organs in the pelvic region. By looking closely at the ultrasound, an experienced clinician can recognize the telltale signs of PID, like swollen fallopian tubes.

In difficult cases, a laparoscopic exploration may be a useful diagnostic procedure. In a laparoscopy, the doctor makes a small incision in the abdomen near the navel and inserts a thin tube with a tiny light and camera. The camera records images that can be viewed on a computer screen. The laparoscope also allows the doctor to use special instruments to take small tissue samples from the pelvic organs for laboratory testing. Laboratory technicians can study the samples and the images to determine what exactly is wrong. If it's PID, then they can figure out how far the disease has progressed.

## TREATMENT

Fortunately, most cases of PID can be treated effectively with antibiotics. Antibiotics are drugs that target bacteria. While antibiotics will stop PID in its tracks, they won't

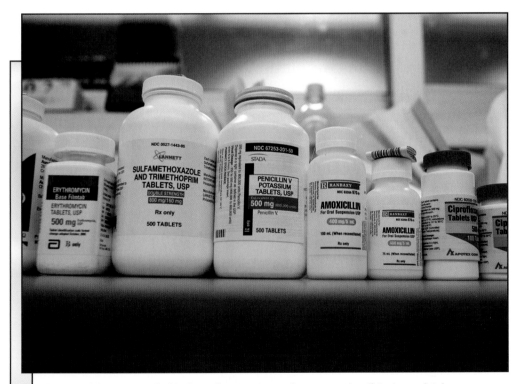

Pictured here is a shelf of antibiotics in a pharmacy. Antibiotics, which target bacteria, are an effective medical treatment for PID.

reverse any damage that has been done already. This is why it's so important to seek care right away, at the first sign of PID. The earlier that antibiotics are administered, the less damage may be done to the reproductive organs. Delaying treatment until it's too late may result in infertility or future ectopic pregnancies.

Antibiotics may be administered orally or by injection. In most cases, the first approach is oral antibiotics. Certain antibiotics are not as effective as others when it comes to targeting specific types of bacteria, so it's common to prescribe at least two different antibiotics for treatment. The idea is to cast as wide a net as possible to make sure the culprit is destroyed. A course of antibiotics should be followed through to completion, even if symptoms disappear. This will ensure that there are no surviving organisms lying in wait to come back again.

A few days after antibiotics are administered, the woman returns to her health care provider for a follow-up exam. If it turns out that oral antibiotics were not effective, then the treating physician may decide to try intravenous antibiotics—antibiotics administered by injection. If this is the case, then hospitalization may be necessary.

There are several other reasons why hospitalization may be recommended. If a woman with PID is pregnant, then doctors may wish to monitor the fetus very closely to ensure that it is healthy and there are no complications. If the patient has severe nausea and is vomiting a lot, then she may need intravenous fluids in order to stay hydrated. Similarly, continuous high fever is dangerous and may be treated best in the hospital. Also, if an abscess is found in the fallopian tube or in an ovary, then surgery may be necessary. Surgery may also be the only way to remove painful scar tissue. And, finally, the health care provider may decide that continuous monitoring is necessary to ensure that the symptoms are not in fact due to something other than PID, like appendicitis.

## OTHER TREATMENT ISSUES

When a woman is treated for PID, her sex partner (or partners) should also be treated, even if there is no sign of infection. A course of antibiotics to destroy any potentially harmful bacteria is typically administered to all sex partners. Sexual activity during treatment may be dangerous and is not recommended. Until all partners have been treated and the disease is completely gone, there is always a chance that it could spread to others.

Finally, it's important to maintain a good diet during treatment. Eating plenty of fruits and vegetables rich in vitamins and minerals will help the body stay strong as it fights the disease. Antibiotics, although extremely important when it comes to treating PID, tend to wear the body down and reduce natural beneficial bacteria as well as the harmful bacteria. A healthy diet can help counteract some of the unwanted effects of antibiotics.

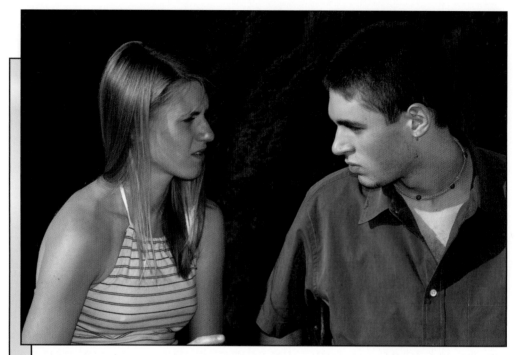

Individuals with a positive diagnosis for PID owe it to their sexual partners to tell them the news. Those partners should then go to a doctor for testing.

## ALTERNATIVE TREATMENTS

Because antibiotics target the pathogenic bacteria responsible for PID, they are universally recommended when it comes to treating the disease. Still, there is a place for adjunct (additional) alternative therapies in PID treatment. Used in combination with antibiotics, such therapies can be very beneficial. Used alone, however, they will not cure the infections that cause PID.

Taking nutritional supplements is one approach. Supplements can provide a boost in the vitamins and minerals the body needs to maintain good health, especially if a woman is having trouble getting adequate nutrition from her diet alone. Supplements, when taken according to recommendations, help guarantee that all nutritional needs are met.

Some women with PID seek herbal treatments for the disease. Derived from plants, herbal remedies, including echinacea, goldenseal, and calendula, are thought to be beneficial when it comes to fighting pathogenic microbes. It has also been said that a warm herbal wrap placed over the lower abdomen can improve circulation and encourage the body's natural healing processes.

Other alternative treatments include homeopathy, acupressure, massage, and acupuncture. These treatments are typically associated with a more holistic approach to medicine. Experienced practitioners in these disciplines consider the needs of the entire body during treatment. By looking at the body as a whole, they seek to restore balance that can improve and maintain one's health over time.

## Ten Great Questions to Ask Your Doctor

1. Does having PID mean I can never have children?

2. How can I keep myself from getting PID?

3. How do I prevent spreading the diseases that cause PID to other people?

4. Are there any signs or symptoms of PID that I should be especially aware of?

5. Can I still date if I have PID?

6. If I have PID, how long will it be before I'm cured?

7. How do you treat PID?

8. Should I be tested for STDs?

9. What should I tell my partner?

10. Am I at a greater risk of future PID infections if I'm infected now?

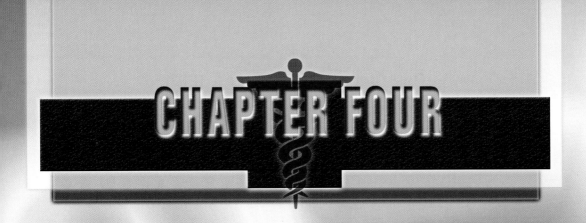

# CHAPTER FOUR

# Coping with PID

The first means of dealing with pelvic inflammatory disease is through immediate treatment. Treatment always includes antibiotics and may also include, depending on the patient, counseling, pain medication, and surgery.

Unfortunately, many women continue to experience both physical and emotional PID-related pain even when treatment is done. For these women, it's important to learn ways to cope with any long-lasting effects of the disease so that they may continue to live happy lives.

## COPING WITH PHYSICAL PROBLEMS

The most common problem among those with PID is pain. Pain in the pelvic region may not go away even after the disease itself is cured. This is because scar tissue may still be present. Like sandpaper on the skin, scar tissue can cause severe irritation.

To reduce the pain, a doctor might prescribe medications. Acupuncture, too, may be effective at reducing pain. Others might find help through alternative means—taking certain herbs, practicing meditation or yoga, or receiving hypnotherapy, for example.

A woman who undergoes surgery as part of her treatment for PID will require time to rest and recover. Teenagers with PID may miss a few days of school because of treatment. For them, it's important to talk to teachers ahead of time about the potential for missed assignments and ways they can make them up.

## EMOTIONAL ISSUES

It's common for those with PID to find it emotionally challenging to deal with. They may wonder why it was they, and not someone else, who had to get the disease in the first place. They may blame themselves for the disease, or they might blame others, including people who really have nothing to do with it. They may feel depressed because they've become—or fear becoming—infertile, because they're suffering from chronic pain, or because they're embarrassed about their situation. There are numerous reasons why a woman with PID might feel emotionally ill.

It's important that people with PID talk about their feelings with those around them—their friends, family, and health care providers. Friends and professionals alike can help steer them back on course and hopefully help them feel better about themselves.

Teens with PID face particular emotional challenges. They may feel shame around their classmates, embarrassed to have come down with a disease that is often associated with sexual promiscuity (having more than one sex partner). For teens with PID, it may help to talk with a counselor at school. He or she can provide advice and encouragement even at the worst of times.

Ultimately, it's important to understand that PID is something that many women have successfully overcome. There are others with PID, and many share the same pain, stress, and discomfort that commonly come with the

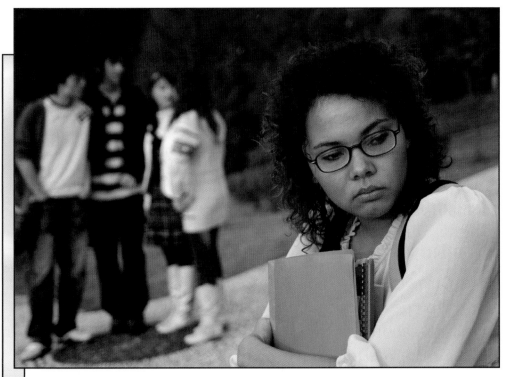

The emotional challenges associated with PID may be just as difficult to deal with as the physical effects of the disease.

disease. They all work their way through it. It just takes time, perseverance, and acceptance.

## SUPPORT GROUPS AND HOTLINES

One of the quickest ways to get help, at least in the beginning, is by calling a free hotline. Two groups that provide hotlines with information about STDs and PID are the American Social Health Association [(800) 227-8922] and the U.S. Department of Health and Human Services' Womenshealth.gov [(800) 994-9662].

Hotlines may be a good resource for locating PID support groups. One may also find support groups by inquiring at health clinics, checking the phone book, and searching online. Support groups are small gatherings of people sharing similar challenges. A PID support group will probably include women currently struggling with PID, as well as women who have fully recovered. There might even be men present. Support group meetings are a great place to go to find compassionate friends when it seems like no one else understands.

## HELPING OTHERS

There are ways for people who don't have PID to help those who do. A woman with PID may like having a person to talk to—about her feelings, about regrets or misgivings, or as a resource for information.

You can be a great help just by being a good and patient listener. By listening, you show you care. And, sometimes,

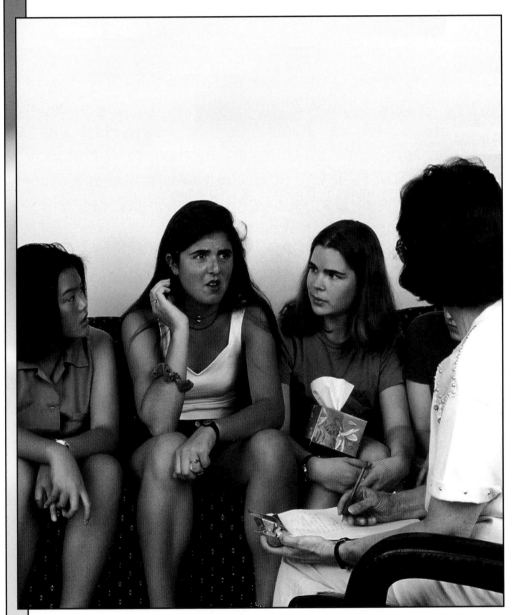

Attending a support group can help you to work through emotional issues related to PID. Other women in the group are probably facing the same challenges.

that's all a person with PID really wants—a friend who cares about her and lets her know that she's not alone.

If a teen with PID must miss school because of pain, a doctor's visit, surgery, or for any other reason, you can help by talking to her teachers, collecting assignments, and taking notes. Help her avoid falling behind in class and you'll do her a great favor. You don't have to tell anyone your friend has PID. It's important to maintain confidentiality when helping anyone with any medical issues. It's up to her if she wants others to know.

If you know of a local resource—a reproductive health clinic, a good doctor—that might be of help to a friend with PID, then tell her about it. Share any connections that you might have. Do you know someone else who has had PID and who might offer to talk? Ask your parents; maybe they know a friend who has recovered from the disease.

## Myths and Facts

**MYTH:** IUDs cause PID.

**FACT:** IUDs do not cause PID. It's the insertion of the IUD in the presence of bacteria that is potentially dangerous. If PID-causing bacteria are present in the woman's lower genital tract at insertion, then there is risk that the IUD will push the bacteria farther up, encouraging the development of PID. Medical experts therefore recommend that women who use IUDs be evaluated for bacterial infection in a follow-up visit after the initial IUD insertion. A woman with active PID should not use an IUD.

**MYTH:** Use of birth control pills provides protection against STDs and, therefore, PID.

**FACT:** Hormonal contraceptives, like birth control pills, do reduce the risk of unplanned pregnancy. In fact, studies have shown birth control pills to be up to 99 percent effective. However, the only way to reduce the risk of contracting an STD during sex is through use of a barrier-style male or female condom. Condoms help prevent the spread of STDs such as chlamydia and gonorrhea—two diseases shown to drastically increase a woman's risk for PID. Some studies suggest birth control pills may stimulate the body to produce thicker-than-normal cervical mucus, which would help protect against PID by making it more difficult for bacteria to pass into the uterus.

**MYTH:** A woman doesn't have PID if she shows no signs or symptoms.

**FACT:** Many women with PID are asymptomatic (showing no symptoms of the disease). The risk in asymptomatic women is that damage may occur without their knowledge. Women who believe they may have been exposed to a sexually transmitted disease should go to their health care provider for testing. Early detection of PID-causing bacteria in the genital tract is the key to containing the disease.

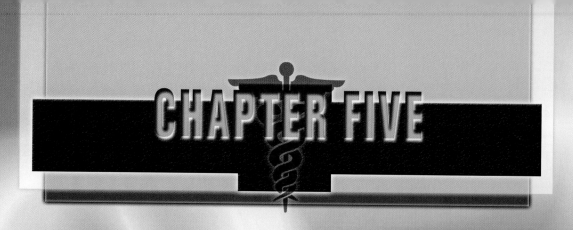

# CHAPTER FIVE

# PID and the Future

How will the story of PID change five, ten, or twenty years from now? Will PID still be the most common complication suffered by women with STDs? Or, will it be a thing of the past—a disease for the record books, never to be heard from again?

Well, it's hard to be optimistic when it comes to wiping out pelvic inflammatory disease for good. The world population continues to boom, and more and more people crowd into smaller and smaller spaces. So, it stands to reason that sexually transmitted diseases, especially, will become harder to control. It may be a difficult future, at least when it comes to PID. It certainly doesn't have to be, though.

## MEDICAL ADVANCES

PID, as you know, can be caused by many different bacteria. And the best way to fight these bacteria is with appropriate antibiotics. The thing about antibiotics and bacteria is that the more often a certain strain of bacteria is exposed to a specific antibiotic, the more likely it will develop resistance to that antibiotic. Over time, that is, older antibiotics become useless. Researchers then have to develop new antibiotics.

To stay ahead of the game, scientists are constantly looking for new antibiotics that may prove more effective than their predecessors, or that can at least take their

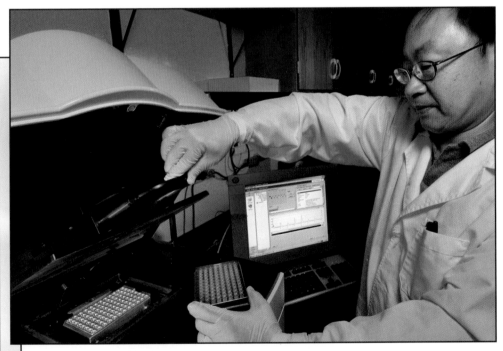

Laboratory researchers worldwide are looking for better ways to treat sexually transmitted diseases. This microbiologist is conducting an experiment using different types of *Chlamydia* bacteria.

place when the time comes. Every year, billions of dollars are spent in medical research looking for ways to combat STDs, PID, and other diseases. This number will continue to grow. Modern medicine is constantly evolving, so chances are good that there will be new treatments—maybe even a cure—in the future.

## STD RESEARCH

Social workers, the medical community, and others are working hard in the war on STDs, but the key to fighting STDs has been, and always will be, prevention. Better prevention comes with better education, increased use of STD-blocking contraceptives, and improved screening. Better sex education is needed in schools, with a focus on abstinence as well as on barrier contraception with condoms. Comprehensive sex ed, which is gradually becoming more common, should arm students with all the knowledge they need to make safer sex a reality—if they choose to have sex at all. That, in turn, should lead to a decrease in STDs and a related decrease in PID.

STD screening is another approach that many medical professionals are trying to improve. Affordable (and sometimes free) clinics for poorer women are becoming more common in urban areas and in developing countries, where STDs are common. These clinics offer a means to screen for STDs. As more women learn of these clinics and drop in for testing, STD incidence should decrease.

## THINKING AHEAD

People who take STDs and PID seriously must consider their own place in the equation. And to do that, they need to have an honest talk about sex. The world is full of people, images, and advertisements depicting sex as exciting and stylish, something everyone is doing all the time. It's everywhere you look: suggestive poses, pouted lips,

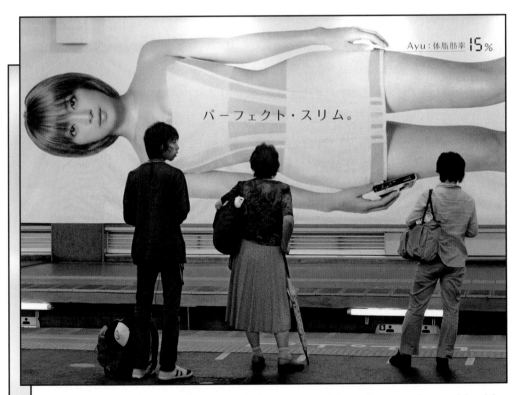

Don't let the media and advertisers influence your ideas about good sexual health. Sex is not all fun and games, and sexy models with perfect faces and bodies are not the norm.

beautiful half-naked people modeling underwear or just driving trendy cars. It is in the movies, music, and magazines, and on television and the Internet. Many teens see these images and wonder if something's wrong with them. Why, they wonder, is everyone having sex but me?

If you've ever wondered about the disconnect between the media's portrayal of sex and your own life, you're not alone. Short and simple, sex sells. It sells clothing, motorcycles, computers, kitchen utensils—you name it. A sexy model can make even the ugliest outfit jump off the shelves.

It would be easy to think that you're the only one in the world not having sex. Or, if you're thinking about having sex, it makes you think that you should jump right into it without a second thought. And if you are having sex, it may make you think that you're not having enough of it.

Are all those images realistic? Are the friends and acquaintances you know in everyday life as sex-crazed as the rock stars, movie stars, and other celebrities on TMZ.com are made out to be? Although it may be difficult at this time, don't let it get to you. Live your own life. Take your time. And don't give in to the pressure. Most people choose for themselves when it's time to start having sex. They have sex when they're ready, with the right person, when they're informed about potential consequences. It's important to educate yourself about sex, sexuality, and sexual health and to make informed, smart decisions when it comes to your personal sex life.

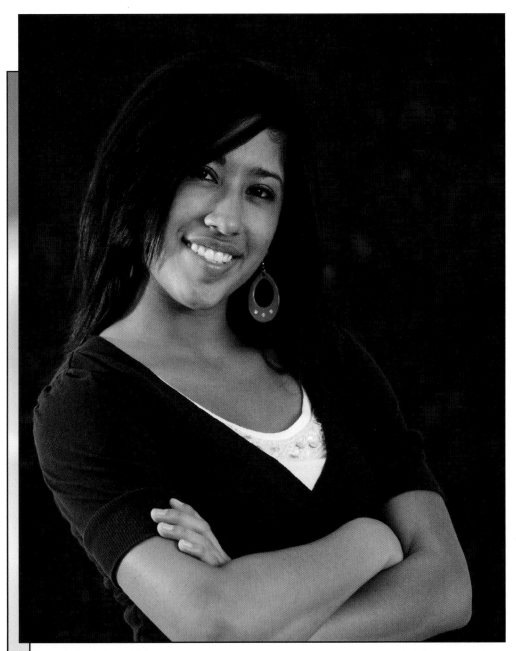

Be smart and be yourself. That's the simple solution to living a happy, healthy life in today's complicated world.

The bottom line is that sex is personal. Everything about it is entirely up to you.

That said, there are situations where making an informed decision about sex is extremely difficult. In the heat of the moment, it's easy to dive right in, forgetting everything you've learned about STDs and unwanted pregnancies. That's passion. It's an overwhelming force. It can shut off your brain—if you let it.

You don't have to, though. If you sharpen your communication skills, goal-setting skills, and decision-making skills, you won't find yourself in situations like that. You can prevent them from happening in the first place. With the right attitude, you can do anything—or, even better, prevent anything.

Maintaining good sexual health is just like maintaining good physical health. To stay physically healthy, you eat a good diet. You exercise. You try to stay balanced in life, with school, work, play, and relationships.

Good sexual health also requires effort. You can begin by being educated. Understand the importance of safer sex. Know how to recognize and avoid STDs. Know the risks. Education is easy. Take a sex ed class. Read books. Talk to older friends. Ask your doctor for more information. Being educated lets you make informed decisions. Make the right decisions, based on the facts at hand, and your problems will be few and far between. You won't have sex with the wrong person. You won't regret your actions.

## Ten Facts About PID

1. Every year, there are more than nineteen million new cases of STDs in the United States.
2. Every year, one in four teens contracts an STD.
3. Almost half of all new STDs occur among people aged fifteen to twenty-four.
4. There are almost three million new cases of chlamydia every year in the United States.
5. PID is responsible for at least 15 percent of infertility cases among U.S. women.
6. Nearly one million American women develop PID every year.
7. An estimated one in eight sexually active adolescent girls develops PID before the age of twenty.
8. Among women treated for PID each year in the United States, at least 200,000 require hospitalization.
9. Bacteria associated with the STDs chlamydia and gonorrhea are the leading causes of PID.
10. Women who have had repeated episodes of PID are at increased risk of infertility.

One way to always make good decisions is by creating a list of goals. Write them out. Do you want to go to college? Are you interested in a certain career? Are you hoping to make a varsity team? Keep those goals in mind when it looks like sex might get in the way. Weigh the risks. Is a one-night stand really in your best interest? Is sex worth it at this stage in the game?

The most important thing you can do for good sexual health is be a great communicator. The one thing about sex is, it's entirely between you and your partner. You need to know how to talk. Be open with each other. If you're thinking about having sex for the first time, then hash it out together. What are your reasons? Are you doing it for yourselves or because you feel pressure? Would it be better to wait?

# GLOSSARY

**abdomen**  The belly; it contains all anatomical structures between the chest and the pelvis.

**abstinence**  Refraining from sexual activity.

**abstinent**  Not sexually active.

**AIDS (acquired immunodeficiency syndrome)**  Illness caused by infection with human immunodeficiency virus (HIV).

**bacteria**  Microscopic organisms that can live in the human body and be either beneficial or harmful.

**barrier-type birth control**  Male or female condom designed to reduce the risk of pregnancy and protect against sexually transmitted diseases.

**cervix**  Narrow portion of the uterus that provides a connection between it and the vagina.

**chlamydia**  Sexually transmitted disease known to be a leading cause of PID.

**chronic**  Long-term and persistent.

**douche**  Device used to flush water into the vagina for cleansing.

**fallopian tubes**  In female anatomy, two narrow tubes providing a passageway for ova as they travel between the ovaries and the uterus.

**genital tract**  Reproductive tract.

**gonorrhea**  Sexually transmitted disease known to be a leading cause of PID.

**hypnotherapy**  Treatment of disease by hypnotism.

**infertile**  Unable to have children.

**inflammation**  Reaction to infection that includes swelling, redness, and irritation.

**intravenous**  Entering by way of a vein.

**IUD**  Intrauterine device.

**microorganism**  Organism that can be seen only with a microscope.

**ovaries**  Female reproductive organs where eggs are produced.

**ovum**  Egg (pl., ova).

**pathogenic**  Disease-causing.

**pelvis**  Ring-shaped region of the skeleton located at the base of the spine; part of the lower abdomen and location of the reproductive tract.

**STD**  Sexually transmitted disease.

**uterus**  Also known as the womb; a major female reproductive organ that houses the developing fetus during pregnancy.

**UTI**  Urinary tract infection.

**vagina**  Tubular female anatomical structure that provides a passageway between the exterior of the body and the uterus.

# FOR MORE INFORMATION

American College of Obstetricians and
    Gynecologists (ACOG)
409 12th Street SW, P.O. Box 96920
Washington, DC 20090-6920
(202) 638-5577
Web site: http://www.acog.org
Founded in 1951, the ACOG is a leading group of
    professionals providing health care for women.

American Social Health Association
P.O. Box 13827
Research Triangle Park, NC 27709
(919) 361-8400
Web site: http://www.ashastd.org
This nonprofit organization devoted to public health is an
    authority on sexually transmitted disease information.

BC Centre for Disease Control
655 West 12th Avenue
Vancouver, BC V5Z 4R4
Canada
(604) 660-2090

Web site: http://www.bccdc.org

The BC Centre for Disease Control is a Canadian agency focusing on preventing and controlling communicable diseases.

Health Canada

Address Locator 0900C2

Ottawa, ON K1A 0K9

Canada

(866) 225-0709

Web site: http://www.hc-sc.gc.ca

Health Canada is the country's federal agency responsible for helping citizens maintain and improve their health.

National Institute of Allergy and Infectious Diseases (NIAID)

NIAID Office of Communications and Government Relations

6610 Rockledge Drive, MSC 6612

Bethesda, MD 20892-6612

(866) 284-4107

TDD: (800) 877-8339 (for hearing impaired)

Web site: http://www3.niaid.nih.gov

NIAID conducts and supports research to better understand, treat, and ultimately prevent infectious, immunologic, and allergic diseases.

National Institutes of Health

9000 Rockville Pike

Bethesda, MD 20892

(301) 496-4000

Web site: http://www.nih.gov

Part of the U.S. Department of Health and Human
Services, the NIH is the primary federal agency for
conducting and supporting medical research, including
studies on children's and teen's health.

U.S. Centers for Disease Control and Prevention (CDC)

1600 Clifton Road

Atlanta, GA 30333

(800) CDC-INFO (232-4636)

Web site: http://www.cdc.gov/std

The CDC is the federal resource for information on all
types of diseases and health-related issues.

## WEB SITES

Due to the changing nature of Internet links, Rosen
Publishing has developed an online list of Web sites
related to the subject of this book. This site is updated
regularly. Please use this link to access the list:

http://www.rosenlinks.com/lsh/pid

# FOR FURTHER READING

Bell, Ruth. *Changing Bodies, Changing Lives*. New York, NY: Three Rivers Press, 1998.

Breguet, Amy. *Chlamydia* (The Library of Sexual Health). New York, NY: Rosen Publishing Group, 2006.

Brynie, Faith Hickman. *101 Questions About Sex and Sexuality*. Minneapolis, MN: Twenty-First Century Books, 2003.

Hunter, Miranda, and William Hunter. *Staying Safe: A Teen's Guide to Sexually Transmitted Diseases*. Broomall, PA: Mason Crest, 2004.

Hyde, Margaret O., and Elizabeth H. Forsyth. *Safe Sex 101: An Overview for Teens*. Minneapolis, MN: Twenty-First Century Books, 2006.

O'Donnell, Judith A. *Pelvic Inflammatory Disease*. New York, NY: Chelsea House, 2006.

Parker, Steve. *The Reproductive System: Injury, Illness and Health*. Chicago, IL: Heinemann Library, 2004.

Perkins, Stephanie C. *Making Smart Choices About Sexual Activity*. New York, NY: Rosen Publishing Group, 2008.

Shoquist, Jennifer, and Diane Stafford. *The Encyclopedia of Sexually Transmitted Diseases* (Facts On File Library of Health and Living). New York, NY: Facts On File, Inc., 2004.

Stanley, Deborah A. *Sexual Health Information for Teens:
    Health Tips About Sexual Development, Human
    Reproduction, and Sexually Transmitted Diseases.*
    Detroit, MI: Omnigraphics, Inc., 2003.

Winters, Adam. *Syphilis* (The Library of Sexual Health).
    New York, NY: Rosen Publishing Group, 2006.

Woods, Samuel G. *Everything You Need to Know About
    STD.* (Need to Know Library). New York, NY: Rosen
    Publishing Group, 2000.

Yancey, Diane. *STDs: What You Don't Know Can Hurt You.*
    Minneapolis, MN: Twenty-First Century Books, 2002.

# BIBLIOGRAPHY

American Social Health Association. "STD/STI Statistics."
    October 2006. Retrieved January 28, 2008 (http://
    www.ashastd.org/learn/learn_statistics.cfm).

Campbell, Neil, and Jane Reece. *Biology*. 5th ed. Menlo
    Park, CA: Benjamin/Cummings, 1999.

Contraception Online. "Sexually Transmitted Infections,
    Risk of HIV Infection, and Condoms: What You Need
    to Know." March 2007. Retrieved January 31, 2008
    (http://www.contraceptiononline.org/contrareport/
    pdfs/07_02_pu.pdf).

Encyclopedia of Alternative Medicine. "Pelvic Inflammatory
    Disease." 2007. Retrieved January 30, 2008 (http://
    findarticles.com/p/articles/mi_g2603/is_0005/ai_
    2603000581).

Ganong, William. *Review of Medical Physiology*. 19th ed.
    Stamford, CT: Appleton & Lange, 1999.

Medline Plus. "Pelvic Inflammatory Disease." September
    2006. Retrieved January 13, 2008 (http://www.nlm.
    nih.gov/medlineplus/ency/article/000888.htm).

National Institute of Allergy and Infectious Diseases.
    "Pelvic Inflammatory Disease." November 2006.
    Retrieved January 28, 2008 (http://www3.niaid.nih.
    gov/healthscience/healthtopics/pelvic/default.htm).

## BIBLIOGRAPHY

U.S. Centers for Disease Control and Prevention. "Pelvic
   Inflammatory Disease—CDC Fact Sheet." December
   2007. Retrieved January 28, 2008 (http://www.cdc.
   gov/std/PID/STDFact-PID.htm).
WebMD. "Women's Health: Your Guide to Pelvic
   Inflammatory Disease, PID." Retrieved January 31,
   2008 (http://women.webmd.com/sexual-health-your-
   guide-to-pelvic-inflammatory-disease).

# INDEX

## ABOUT THE AUTHOR

Michael R. Wilson is a health and science writer. He has written on many health- and biology-related topics for Rosen Publishing, including the human brain, the cardiopulmonary system, and genetics.

## PHOTO CREDITS

Cover © www.istockphoto.com; p. 1 © Scott Bodell/Getty Images; p. 4 www.istockphoto.com/ericsphotography, 4 (silhouette) © www.istockphoto.com/jamesbenet; p. 5 © David Young-Wolff/Photo Edit; p. 9 © CNRI/Photo Researchers; p. 10 © www.istockphoto.com/Thomas Paschke; p. 15 © VOISIN/Photo Researchers; pp. 20, 31 © Getty Images; p. 24 © www.istockphoto.com/Sheryl Griffin; p. 26 © Bob Pardue/Alamy; p. 29 © Adam Gault/Photo Researchers; p. 34 © Ellen Senisi/The Image Works; p. 39 © www.istockphoto.com/Robert Churchill; p. 41 © Michael Newman/Photo Edit; p. 45 Hsi Liu, Ph.D., MBA, James Gathany/CDC; p. 47 © AF/Getty Images; p. 49 © www.istockphoto.com/Jason Stephen; back cover (top to bottom) 3D4Medical.com/Getty Images, © www.istockphoto.com/Luis Carlos Torres, © www.istockphoto.com/Kiyoshi Takahase Segundo, CDC, © www.istockphoto.com/Amanda Rohde, Scott Bodell/Photodisc/Getty Images.

**Designer:** Nelson Sá; **Editor:** Christopher Roberts
**Photo Researcher:** Marty Levick

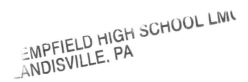